Heart Healthy Smoothies

125 Delicious Recipes
for Natural Reduction and
Control of High Blood Pressure

Clyde Verhine

TABLE OF CONTENTS

TABLE OF CONTENTS (CONTINUED)

Chapter 1
Why I Wrote This Book

"The doctor of the future will give no medicine, but will interest his patients in the care of the human frame, in diet and in the cause and prevention of disease." ~ *Thomas Edison*

In my book High Blood Pressure and You - The Effects of High Blood Pressure, Prescription Drug Side Effects, and Natural Ways To Reduce And Control High Blood Pressure , I discuss in detail natural ways to reduce and control high blood pressure. One chapter of that book ("What To Eat") discusses why one of the most important factors in controlling blood pressure is having a healthy and balanced diet that provides the nutrients needed to maintain healthy blood pressure levels. Potassium, magnesium, and calcium are identified as the most important minerals needed for good blood pressure management. Also very important are Coenzyme Q10, Omega-3 fatty acids, Vitamin B-6, and Vitamin C. If you want to maintain, reduce, and/or control your blood pressure, you need to concentrate on items in your diet that will supply these minerals, vitamins, and other nutrients that are critical in blood pressure control. In that chapter of my other book, I identified and described in more detail the foods that contain these needed dietary components and ways to increase these items in your diet. One suggestion in the book is about how to easily increase your consumption by to using your blender to make smoothies from the foods that provide the most benefits for heart health and blood pressure control.

I decided that a book of smoothie recipes from the identified most beneficial dietary items would be helpful to those who are serious about keeping their blood pressure under control using natural methods (with or without prescription medication). Not only is drinking smoothies from these recipes healthy, the smoothies are also easy to make and delicious.

This book is intended to be a companion to my book High Blood Pressure and You - The Effects of High Blood Pressure, Prescription Drug Side Effects, and Natural Ways To Reduce And Control High Blood Pressure which is also available as a Kindle or printed version on Amazon.

~~~ ~~~ ~~~ ~~~ ~~~

Chapter 2
About High Blood Pressure

Every adult needs to be aware of the potential that they have high blood pressure. Over 1 in 5 Americans that have high blood pressure are not aware of it. 1 in 3 adults today have this condition and the older you are the greater your chances of having this potentially deadly condition.

High blood pressure is known as the "Silent Killer" because there is usually no symptoms to alert a person until that person has a stroke or heart attack. High blood pressure contributes to over 1000 deaths in the US every day.

One in three adults in America today have high blood pressure, and for those older than age 60, the number is over six in ten. There are millions of Americans who have been diagnosed with high blood pressure and put on medication but still do not have their blood pressure under control. Many of the people who take these medications are not aware of the risks and potential side effects of the drug(s) they are taking.

Usually there is no one specific cause identifiable for high blood pressure (also called primary hypertension). However, there are several factors known to increase the risk. One of these is a diet that include a lot of highly processed convenience foods which usually contain high amounts of sodium and artificial preservatives, and are lacking in the vitamins and minerals needed for blood pressure control.

Fortunately, treatment for high blood isn't limited to just prescription drugs. If you reduce you blood pressure by using natural methods to maintain a healthy lifestyle, you might postpone, reduce or even eliminate the need for prescription medication. One of the natural methods of lowering blood pressure (whether you take prescriptions for it or not) is to get the proper nutrients (in the needed amounts) from your diet. Drinking the smoothies from the recipes in this book will help make sure you are getting these nutrients.

~~~ ~~~ ~~~ ~~~ ~~~

Chapter 3
Blood Pressure And Smoothies

The American Heart Association recommends nine servings (about 4.5 cups) of fruits and vegetables be eaten every day. The best way to get the nutrients you need are to eat the vegetables and fruits, but is is often hard to get these recommended servings just by eating. Juicing or blending vegetables and fruits are an alternative that can be used to easily increase consumption. There is a however a difference between juicing and blending.

A juicer gives you a nutrient rich liquid of vegetables and fruits without the fiber or pulp. Drinking the liquid juice gives you a faster release and absorption of the nutrients but since many nutrients of the fruits and vegetables are found in the fiber and pulp, you will not get as much of the food's nutrients as you would using a blending method. Juicing can be more expensive because of the equipment needed and the amount of juice that can be obtained relative to the volume of the produce

A better choice to get the most of the nutrients found in dietary items is to blend them. Blenders are more common and usually a less expensive appliance than a juicer. In addition, whatever you put in the blender is what you will get to drink. Blended vegetables and fruits which gives a more filling drink. Blended items also give a slower, more sustained release of food's nutrients. Consuming the fiber and pulp content helps reduce overeating because it is more filling, plus it is also helpful in the digestive process Another plus in using a blender is that you can add other things like nuts, seeds, milk, and/or yogurt to increase your intake of additional minerals, vitamins, and healthy fats. Herbs, spices and/or honey can also be added to enhance the taste of your blended drink.

These blended drinks are sometimes called smoothies. The aim of this book is to provide a selection of recipes for smoothies made from the food items that have been identified as being the most beneficial for reducing and controlling high blood pressure. In this book you will find 125 recipes for heart healthy smoothies. To help insure that these are recipes you can use, I also tried to keep them as simple as possible and not to include any exotic or hard to find items.

~~~ ~~~ ~~~ ~~~ ~~~

Chapter 4
About Blending and The Recipes

* About the blender:

The best blenders for making smoothies have a powerful motor (500+ watts) with variable speed settings, a heavy stable base (preferable made of metal), a lid that fits tightly and will not come off during the blending process, and one that has a base and container that are easily cleaned.

* Comments for all recipes:

For recipes that call for water, ice, or other liquids, you can add more or less depending on how thick and/or how cold you want to make your smoothie. If you don't want the chilled versions, substitute thawed or fresh for frozen ingredients listed in the recipe.

Add more of a liquid ingredient for a thinner smoothie, add less for thicker. I will put a (+-) beside the water, ice, other variable liquid ingredient(s) amount in the recipe. I will also put a (+-) beside recipe ingredients that should be added according to your individual tastes.

The amount of smoothie each recipe will make varies with each recipe making between 2 to 4 smoothies depending on the size of your smoothie glass. Since blender containers vary in amount they can hold, each recipe can be adjusted by proportionately increasing or decreasing the amounts indicated on each recipe to achieve the desired serving size. Most of these recipes were based on a blender that holds 4 cups of blended liquid. If you make more than you can drink at once, and you want to save it for later, be sure to store your blended smoothie in the refrigerator. The smoothie will keep and remain fresh tasting when stored in a sealed container in the refrigerator for 1 or 2 days.

If the recipe calls for ice or ice cubes and unless you have a very powerful blender, it is best to crush the ice before putting it into the blender. This reduces wear on your blender motor and blades. You can make your own crushed ice by placing ice cubes in a plastic bag, wrap the bag in a cloth towel, place the towel/bag on a cutting board, and "crush" the ice with a wooden mallet, rolling pin, meat tenderizing mallet, etc..

If a recipe calls for milk and you are lactose intolerant, just substitute your favorite rice milk, nut milk (like almond or hazelnut milk), soy milk, coconut milk, etc...

* Directions for all recipes:

Unless otherwise noted, place all ingredients in the recipe into blender except water and ice. To lessen wear on the blender, make sure there is some liquid added before starting the process. Begin with lesser amounts of items marked (+-) than called for on the recipes. After adding some of the liquid ingredients in the blender, put the softer items in first followed by harder items, followed by any frozen items, followed by any leafy greens, and last more of the liquid items.

Once the ingredients are in place in the blender container, place the top securely on the blender, and then start the blender. Let it run until all items are fully blended.

After blending, stop the blender, remove the top, and test consistency and taste. If needed, stir to move any chunks that may not have fully blended, add additional water, ice, and/or other items. Put the top back on the blender and restart. Repeat this last step until you are comfortable with the taste and the liquid consistency of the blended smoothie.

* Since every person's tastes are different:

You may find the texture of some of the blended raw vegetables to be to course or grainy. In some cases you can cook the vegetables before blending, you might decrease that ingredient and increase another one, or you may find a less grainy substitute. In order to get the most benefits from the blended drinks, it is important that you find flavor combinations that you like. Do not be afraid to experiment and try other combinations of ingredients from the lists of different dietary items on other recipes in this book. Once you find a combination you like, the more likely you are to make and drink it on a regular basis.

Just as in my book <u>High Blood Pressure and You</u>, I have organized these recipes following the sections of that book in these categories: Vegetables, Fruits, Beans, Nuts, Herbs and Spice, and Other.

~~~ ~~~ ~~~ ~~~ ~~~

Chapter 5
Smoothie Recipes - Vegetables

Vegetables contain vitamins and fiber, and many are rich in potassium, calcium, and/or magnesium which work to keep your body and blood pressure in good condition. Canned and frozen vegetables can be comparable to fresh in nutritional values as long as they do not contain added sugars and fats, artificial preservatives, or excessive amounts of added sodium.

Be sure to wash all fresh vegetables thoroughly before blending.

Asparagus

Asparagus is a perennial plant with succulent tall herbaceous stems and flowery foliage. Asparagus is high in anti-inflammatory and antioxidant nutrients. It is also known as a natural diuretic.

* Asparagus / Strawberry / Orange Juice / Milk

~ Asparagus - 6 spears - lightly steamed
~ Strawberries - 3/4 cup - frozen
~ Orange Juice - 3/4 cup - fresh squeezed
~ Milk - 1 3/4 cups - 2% or low-fat
~ Honey - 1 (+-) tablespoon (optional for sweetness)
~ Vanilla Extract - 1 teaspoon
~ Ice - 5 (+-) cubes

Asparagus / Apple / Cantaloupe / Spinach

~ Asparagus - 6 spears - raw or lightly steamed
~ Apple - 1 tart green (Granny Smith) - with peel but cored - sliced
~ Cantaloupe - 1 cup - peeled and cubed
~ Spinach - 1 cup - fresh baby spinach
~ Milk - 1/2 cup - skim or almond
~ Honey - 1 (+-) tablespoon (optional for sweetness)
~ Water - 1/2 (+-) cup
~ Ice - 3 (+-) cubes

Asparagus / Apple / Zucchini / Tomato / Cucumber / Grape / Parsley

~ Asparagus - 6 Spears - raw or lightly steamed
~ Apple - 1 sweet red - with peel but cored - sliced
~ Zucchini - 1 chopped
~ Tomato - 1 large - chopped
~ Cucumber - 1/2 peeled - chopped
~ Grapes - 1 cup seedless - any color
~ Parsley - 1 cup - chopped
~ Water - 1/2 (+-) cup
~ Ice - 3 (+-) cubes

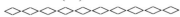

Bok Choy

Bok Choy is loaded with blood pressure reducing potassium, calcium, and magnesium. Bok Choy is a cruciferous vegetable related to cabbage. It looks like Romaine lettuce at the top and large celery on the bottom. Bok choy has a mild flavor and can be eaten raw like celery.

Bok Choy / Banana / Ginger / Mint
~ Bok Choy - 2 cups - leaves and stalks - chopped
~ Banana - 1 - peeled - cut in 1 inch pieces - frozen
~ Ginger Root - 1 inch piece - finely chopped
~ Mint Leaves - 1/2 cup
~ Water - 1 (+-) cup - coconut water or plain

Bok Choy / Orange / Apple / Lemon
~ Bok Choy - 2 cups - leaves and stalks - chopped
~ Orange - 1 large - peeled - segmented - seeds removed
~ Apple - 1 sweet red - with peel but cored - sliced
~ Lemon - 1/2 - juiced - use juice only
~ Water - 1 (+-) cup
~ Ice - 2 (+-) cubes

Bok Choy / Blueberry / Lemon / Ginger
~ Bok Choy - 1 head - baby bok choy - chopped
~ Blueberry - 1 cup - fresh or frozen
~ Lemon - 1/2 - juiced - use juice only
~ Ginger Root - 1 inch piece - finely chopped
~ Parsley - 1/3 cup - chopped
~ Water - 1/2 (+-) cup
~ Ice - 3 (+-) cubes
◇◇◇◇◇◇◇◇◇◇

Broccoli

Broccoli is also a cruciferous vegetable. It is loaded with Vitamin C as well as being rich in other vitamins, minerals, and antioxidants. If you like the taste of broccoli, it is more nutritious if eaten raw. To reduce the grainy texture in the smoothie you may want to lightly steam the broccoli before putting it into the blender.

Broccoli / Blueberry / Strawberry
~ Broccoli - 3/4 cup - chopped - raw or lightly steamed
~ Blueberry - 1 cup - frozen
~ Strawberry - 1/2 cup
~ Juice - 1 cup - cranberry or cranberry/apple
~ Yogurt - 1/2 cup - low fat - unsweetened

Broccoli / Apple / Honey
~ Broccoli - 1 1/2 cups - chopped - raw or lightly steamed
~ Apple - 1 cup - tart green (Granny Smith) - with peel but cored - sliced
~ Honey - 2 (+-) tablespoons
~ Lemon Juice - 4 tablespoons
~ Water - 1 (+-) cup
~ Ice - 1/2 (+-) cup

Broccoli / Banana / Orange
~ Broccoli - 1 cup - chopped - raw or lightly steamed
~ Banana - 1 peeled - cut in 1 inch pieces - frozen
~ Orange - 1 cup - peeled - segmented - seeds removed
~ Milk - 1 cup - 2% or low fat
~ Ice - 4 (+-) cubes

◇◇◇◇◇◇◇◇◇◇

Brussel Sprouts

Brussel sprouts look like miniature cabbages and have a nutty, earthy taste. It is a cruciferous vegetable that is rich in vitamins, minerals, and antioxidants.

Brussel Sprouts / Raspberries / Walnuts
~ Brussel Sprout - 1 1/2 cup - chopped - raw or lightly steamed
~ Raspberries - 1 cups - frozen
~ Walnuts - 1/4 cup - finely chopped
~ Honey - 1 (+-) tablespoon
~ Water - 3/4 (+-) cups
~ Ice - 1/2 (+-) cup

Brussel Sprouts / Cucumber / Apple / Banana
~ Brussel Sprout - 1 cup - chopped - raw or lightly steamed
~ Cucumber - 1 cup - peeled - chopped
~ Apple - 1 sweet red - with peel but cored - sliced
~ Banana - 1 - peeled - cut in 1 inch pieces - frozen
~ Water - 1/2 cup (+-)
~ Ice - 2 cubes (+-)

Brussel Sprouts / Strawberries / Grapes / Almonds
~ Brussel Sprout - 1 cup - chopped - raw or lightly steamed
~ Strawberries - 1/2 cup - fresh or frozen
~ Grapes - 1/2 cup seedless - any color
~ Almonds - 1/4 cup - finely chopped
~ Milk - 1 (+-) cup - 2%, low fat, or almond
~ Vanilla Extract - 1/8 (+-) teaspoon
~ Ice - 3/4 (+-) cup
◇◇◇◇◇◇◇◇◇◇◇

Cabbage

There are many different varieties of cabbage, but for these recipes, the most commonly identified cabbages which are the densely leaved green and red/purple cabbages are used. Cabbage is loaded with the vitamins and minerals needed for high blood pressure control.

Cabbage / Blueberries / Banana
~ Cabbage - 2 cups - red - shredded
~ Blueberries - 1 cup - frozen
~ Banana - 1 - peeled - cut in 1 inch pieces - frozen
~ Yogurt - 1/2 cup - low fat - unsweetened
~ Vanilla Extract - 1/8 (+-) teaspoon
~ Water - 1/4 (+-) cups
~ Ice - 1/2 (+-) cups

Cabbage / Grapes / Mango / Carrot
~ Cabbage - 1 cups - green - shredded
~ Grapes - 1 cup - seedless - any color
~ Mango - 1 cup - chunks - frozen
~ Carrot - 1 large - chopped
~ Water - 1/2 (+-) cup
~ Ice - 2 (+-) cubes

Cabbage / Banana / Blackberry/ Almond
~ Cabbage - 1 cups - green - shredded
~ Banana - 1 - peeled - cut in 1 inch pieces - frozen
~ Blackberries - 1 cup - frozen
~ Almonds - 1/4 cup - chopped
~ Honey - 1 (+-) tablespoon
~ Water - 1 (+-) cups
~ Ice - 1/4 (+-) cups
◇◇◇◇◇◇◇◇◇◇◇◇

Carrot

Carrots are root vegetables rich in beta-carotene (converted by the body into vitamin A) and alpha-carotene. Studies show that diets that are high in carotenoids are associated with lower risks for heart disease. According to a study at Harvard University, people who ate five or more carrots a week are less likely to suffer a stroke than those who eat only one carrot a month or less.

Carrot / Banana / Mango
~ Carrot - 1 cup - baby - chopped
~ Banana - 1 medium - peeled - cut into pieces
~ Mango - 1 cup - chunks - frozen
~ Orange Juice - 1 cup - fresh squeezed
~ Water - 1/4 (+-) cup

Carrot / Orange / Ginger
~ Carrot - 2 cups - chopped
~ Orange - 2 large - peeled - segmented - seeds removed
~ Ginger Root - 3/4 (+-) inch piece - finely chopped
~ Water - 1/4 (+-) cup
~ Ice - 3 (+-) cubes (optional to chill if desired)

Carrot / Spinach / Banana
~ Carrot - 1 cup - peeled - chopped
~ Spinach - 2 (+-) cups - baby spinach leaves
~ Banana - 1 large - peeled - cut into pieces
~ Yogurt - 3/4 cup - low fat - unsweetened
~ Honey - 2 (+-) tablespoons
~ Water - 1/4 (+-) cup
~ Ice - 1/2 (+-) cups
◇◇◇◇◇◇◇◇◇◇◇

Celery

Celery is another vegetable high in anti-inflammatory and antioxidant nutrients. It also contains vitamins A (as beta-carotene) and K, as well as calcium and healthy, natural sodium. You will find that the smaller less fibrous stalks work best to reduce the grainy texture in the smoothie that comes from the celery.

Celery, Apple, Blueberry, Cashew
~ Celery - 1 1/2 cups - trimmed - finely chopped
~ Apple - 1 red - cored - peeled - chopped
~ Blueberry - 1 1/2 cups - frozen
~ Cashew - 4 tablespoons - chopped
~ Water - 3/4 (+-) cup

Celery, Banana, Strawberry, Spinach
~ Celery - 1 1/2 cups - trimmed - finely chopped
~ Banana - 1 medium - peeled - cut into pieces
~ Strawberry - 3/4 cup - frozen
~ Spinach - 2 (+-) cups - baby spinach leaves
~ Water - 1/4 (+-) cup

Celery, Mango, Cucumber
~ Celery - 3/4 cup - trimmed - finely chopped
~ Mango - 1 1/2 cups - chunks - frozen
~ Cucumber - 1 cup - peeled - chopped
~ Basil - 1 (+-) tablespoon - fresh
~ Lemon Juice - 1 (+-) teaspoon - fresh squeezed
~ Water - 3/4 (+-) cup
~ Ice - 1/4 (+-) cup

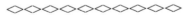

Cauliflower

Cauliflower is another cruciferous vegetable. White is the most common color associated with cauliflower but it also comes in orange, purple, and green. It is a waste when the green leaves of the cauliflower are discarded. The leaves and stems of the cauliflower are edible and contain vital nutrients.

Cauliflower, Strawberry, Grapes
~ Cauliflower - 1 cup - chopped
~ Strawberries - 1 cup - fresh or frozen
~ Grapes - 1 cup - seedless - any color
~ Milk - 1/2 cup - 2% or almond milk
~ Water - 1/2 (+-) cup
~ Ice - 3 (+-) cubes (if chilled drink desired)

Cauliflower, Avocado, Blueberry, Banana
~ Cauliflower - 1 cup - chopped
~ Avocado - 1 fully ripe - halved - pitted - peeled - chopped
~ Blueberry - 2 cup - frozen
~ Banana - 1 large - peeled - cut into pieces
~ Hibiscus Tea - 1 (+-) cup

Cauliflower, Spinach, Carrot, Apple
~ Cauliflower - 1 cup - chopped
~ Spinach - 1 (+-) cups - baby spinach leaves
~ Carrot - 1/2 cup - baby - chopped
~ Apple - 1/2 cup - sweet red - cored - peeled - chopped
~ Pumpkin Seed - 1 tablespoon - chopped
~ Honey - 1 (+-) teaspoon
~ Water - 1/2 (+-) cup
~ Ice - 1/2 (+-) cup
◇◇◇◇◇◇◇◇◇◇◇◇

Cucumber

Even though cucumber is generally referred to as a vegetable, since the cucumber grows from the flower of the plant, the cucumber is technically a fruit. It belongs to the same family as melons and squash. Cucumbers contain anti-inflammatory compounds, powerful antioxidants, and other nutrients essential to natural blood pressure control. Cucumber is also a natural diuretic.

Cucumber / Blueberry
~ Cucumber - 1 1/2 cup - peeled - chopped
~ Blueberry - 1 cup - frozen
~ Yogurt - 1 cup - low fat - unsweetened
~ Honey - 1 tablespoon
~ Lemon Juice - 1 tablespoon
~ Water - 1/2 (+-) cup

Cucumber / Cantaloupe / Watermelon / Leafy Green
~ Cucumber - 1 cup - peeled - chopped
~ Cantaloupe - 1 cup - rind removed - chunks - frozen
~ Watermelon - 1 cup - rind removed - chunks - frozen
~ Leafy Green - 1/2 (+-) cup - Kale or Baby Spinach
~ Lemon Juice - 1 teaspoon
~ Water - 1/2 (+-) cup

Cucumber / Apple / Mint
~ Cucumber - 2 cups - peeled - chopped
~ Apple - 1/3 cup - sweet red - cored - peeled - chopped
~ Apple Juice - 2/3 cup - unsweetened concentrate - frozen - undiluted
~ Mint - 1/4 cup - fresh - chopped
~ Water - 1/4 (+-) cup
~ Ice - 1/2 (+-) cup
◇◇◇◇◇◇◇◇◇◇

Eggplant

The eggplant belongs to the nightshade family of plants so the flowers and leaves are poisonous if eaten in large enough quantities. Eggplants are available in many shapes, sizes and a variety of colors. The best-known variety of eggplant has a deep purple skin. The most common way to eat eggplant is cooked since the raw fruit can sometimes have a bitter taste.

Eggplant / Zucchini / Grapes / Strawberry
~ Eggplant - 1/2 cups - peeled - chopped - boiled - cooled
~ Zucchini - 1/2 cups - peeled - chopped
~ Grapes - 1 cup - purple or red - frozen
~ Strawberry - 1 cup - frozen
~ Vanilla Extract - 1/8 (+-) teaspoon
~ Water - 1/2 (+-) cup

Eggplant / Grapes / Orange Juice
~ Eggplant - 1 1/2 cup - peeled - chopped - boiled - cooled
~ Grapes - 1 1/2 cup - frozen
~ Orange Juice - 1 cup - fresh squeezed

Eggplant / Banana
~ Eggplant - 2 cups - peeled - chopped - boiled - cooled
~ Banana - 1 large - peeled - cut into pieces - frozen
~ Milk - 1 cup - almond milk
~ Honey - 1 (+-) tablespoon
~ Ice - 3 (+-) cubes
◇◇◇◇◇◇◇◇◇◇◇

Fennel

Fennel is a flowering plant species in the carrot family, and all parts of the plant (bulb, stalk, leaves, and seeds) are edible. Fennel has a mild but distinctive licorice flavor and is used in much the same way as celery.

Fennel / Apple / Carrot / Ginger
~ Fennel - 1 cup - bulb only - sliced or chopped
~ Apple - 1 sweet crisp - with skin - cored
~ Carrot - 3/4 cup - peeled - chopped
~ Ginger - 1 tablespoon - fresh peeled - slices
~ Apple Juice - 1 cup - unsweetened
~ Lemon Juice - 1 tablespoon - fresh squeezed

Fennel / Plum / Lemon
~ Fennel - 1 cup - bulb and fronds - chopped
~ Plum - 2 cups - purple plums - pits removed - sliced - frozen
~ Lemon - 1 medium - peeled - seeds removed
~ Water - 1/2 (+-) cup

Fennel / Blackberry / Banana
~ Fennel - 1 cup - bulb only - sliced or chopped
~ Blackberry - 1 cup - frozen
~ Banana - 1 large - peeled - cut into pieces
~ Lemon Juice - 1 tablespoon - fresh squeezed
~ Vanilla Extract - 1/8 (+-) teaspoon
~ Water - 1 (+-) cup

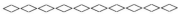

Garlic

Garlic is a vegetable bulb and is a close relative to leeks, chives, and onions. Garlic is generally used as a flavoring ingredient rather than as the main ingredient itself. Garlic contains a substance called allicin which has been shown to have antibacterial, antioxidant, lipid lowering and anti-hypertensive properties.

Garlic / Tomato / Cucumber / Apple / Onion / Leafy Greens
~ Garlic - 2 (+-) cloves - peeled - finely minced
~ Tomato - 3/4 cup - chopped
~ Cucumber - 1/4 cup - peeled - chopped
~ Apple - 1/2 cup - sweet red - cored - peeled - chopped
~ Onion - 1/4 cup - sweet - chopped
~ Celery - 3/4 cup - trimmed - finely chopped
~ Leafy Green - 2 (+-) cups – any variety - chopped
~ Water - 1 1/2 (+-) cups
~ Ice - 1/2 (+-) cup

Garlic / Spinach / Apple / Avocado / Tomato
~ Garlic - 2 (+-) cloves - peeled - finely minced
~ Spinach - 1 cups - baby - chopped
~ Apple - 1/2 cup - sweet red - cored - peeled - chopped
~ Avocado - 1/2 fully ripe - halved - pitted - peeled - chopped
~ Tomato - 1 cup - chopped
~ Water - 3/4 (+-) cups
~ Ice - 1/2 (+-) cup

(Garlic – continued next page)

(Garlic – continued)

Garlic / Bok Choy / Cucumber / Carrot / Lemon / Onion / Tomato
~ Garlic - 2 (+-) cloves - peeled - finely minced
~ Bok Choy - 1 cup - leaves and stalks - chopped
~ Cucumber - 3/4 cup - peeled - chopped
~ Carrot - 1/2 cup - baby - chopped
~ Lemon - 1 medium - peeled - seeds removed
~ Onion - 1/4 cup - red, yellow, white, or sweet - chopped
~ Tomato Juice - 1 cup - low sodium
~ Turmeric - 1/8 (+-) teaspoon
~ Black Pepper - 1/8 (+-) teaspoon
~ Ice - 1/2 (+-) cup
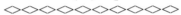

Leafy Greens

Leafy greens provide a major dietary source for heart healthy minerals and vitamins. Arugula, collard greens, kale, mustard greens, Romaine lettuce, spinach, Swiss chard, turnip greens, and watercress are all leafy greens that are high in vitamins and minerals. Leafy greens can be eaten raw, but you get more benefits related to blood pressure when the greens are cooked. The most common and best leafy green choices for blood pressure control are kale, turnip greens, and spinach.

Kale / Banana / Fig / Pistachio

~ Kale - 1 cup - trimmed - chopped - boiled or steamed (5 minutes) - cooled

~ Banana - 1 - peeled - cut in 1 inch pieces - frozen

~ Fig - 1 fresh - halved - (if using dried figs be sure to re-hydrate 1 to 2 hours)

~ Pistachios - 1/2 cup - chopped - (can substitute cashews)

~ Ginger - 1/2 (+-) teaspoon - finely minced

~ Vanilla Extract - 1 (+-) teaspoon

~ Milk - 1 1/2 (+-) cups - 2% or almond milk

~ Ice - 1/2 (+-) cup

Turnip Greens / Mango / Cucumber / Celery / Lemon

~ Turnip Greens - 1 1/2 cups - chopped - boiled or steamed (5 minutes) - cooled

~ Mango - 1 cup - chunks - frozen

~ Cucumber - 1/2 cup - peeled - chopped

~ Celery - 1/2 cup - trimmed - finely chopped

~ Lemon - 1/2 - peeled - seeds removed

~ Basil - 1/4 (+-) cup - chopped

~ Water - 1/2 (+-) cup

~ Ice - 4 (+-) cubes

(Leafy Greens – continued next page ...)

(Leafy Greens – continued ...)

Spinach / Berries / Yogurt / Orange Juice
~ Spinach - 1/2 cup - fresh baby spinach - chopped
~ Mixed Berries - 1 cup - frozen
~ Yogurt - 1 cup - plain - unsweetened
~ Orange Juice - 1 cup - fresh squeezed
~ Water - 1/2 (+-) cup
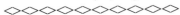

Onion

Even though yellow onions are the most grown, there are over 30 varieties of onions in a variety of sizes, colors, and flavors. Onions are filled with quercetin which is a powerful antioxidant flavonol effective in reducing blood pressure. Both raw or cooked onions are good natural sources of nutrients for blood pressure control, but studies show that raw onions are more effective for reducing high blood pressure.

Onion / Tomato / Carrot / Zucchini
~ Onion - 1/2 cup - sweet - chopped
~ Tomato - 2 cups - chopped
~ Carrot - 1/2 cup - baby - chopped - frozen
~ Zucchini - 1/2 cup - chopped
~ Oregano - 1 teaspoon
~ Basil - 1 teaspoon
~ Vinegar - 1 tablespoon
~ Black Pepper - 1/2 (+-) teaspoon
~ Turmeric - 1/4 (+-) teaspoon
~ Water - 1/2 (+-) cup
~ Ice - 3 (+-) cubes

Onion / Carrot / Apple / Sweet Potato
~ Onion - 3/4 cup - yellow or sweet - chopped
~ Carrot - 1/2 cup - baby - chopped - frozen
~ Apple - 1 cup - sweet red - cored - chopped
~ Sweet Potato - 1 cup - baked - peeled - chopped - cooled
~ Ginger - 1/2 (+-) teaspoon - finely minced
~ Water - 1/2 (+-) cup
~ Ice - 3 (+-) cubes

(Onion – continued next page)

(Onions – continued)

Onion / Cauliflower / Cucumber / Apple / Lemon / Carrot

~ Onion - 1/2 cup - red - chopped
~ Cauliflower - 1 cup - chopped
~ Cucumber - 1/2 cup - peeled - chopped
~ Apple - 1/2 cup - sweet red - cored - peeled - chopped
~ Lemon - 1 medium - peeled - seeds removed
~ Carrot Juice - 1 cup - organic
~ Turmeric - 1/8 (+-) teaspoon
~ Black Pepper - 1/8 (+-) teaspoon
~ Water - 1/2 (+-) cup
~ Ice - 3 (+-) cubes

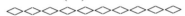

Potato

There are over 100 varieties within the seven categories of potatoes sold in the US. The russet potato (or Idaho potato) is the most common. Because of the potential for gastric problems, it is recommended that potatoes not be eaten raw and uncooked

Potato / Kale / Apple

~ Potato - 1 cups - red - boiled - cooled - peeled - sliced
~ Kale - 1 cup - trimmed - chopped - boiled or steamed (5 minutes) - cooled
~ Apple - 3/4 cup - sweet red - cored - peeled - chopped
~ Lemon - 1 large - juice only
~ Water - 1/2 (+-) cup
~ Ice - 1/2 (+-) cup

Potato / Mango / Milk

~ Potato - 1 cup - russet, white, or yellow - boiled - cooled - peeled - sliced
~ Mango - 1.5 cup - chunks - frozen
~ Milk - 1 cup - 2%
~ Honey - 1 (+-) tablespoon
~ Water - 1/2 (+-) cup
~ Ice - 3 (+-) cubes

Potato / Milk

~ Potato - 1.5 cups - russet, white, or yellow - boiled - cooled - peeled - sliced
~ Milk - 2 cup - coconut, almond, or 2%
~ Cinnamon - 3/4 (+-) teaspoon - ground
~ Nutmeg - 3/4 (+-) teaspoon - ground
~ Honey - 1 (+-) tablespoon
~ Water - 1/2 (+-) cup
~ Ice - 3 (+-) cubes
◇◇◇◇◇◇◇◇◇◇

Potato - Sweet

The sweet potato is a large, sweet tasting, starchy a root vegetable. They are a very good source for beta-carotene (vitamin A), vitamin C, and potassium - all very important for high blood pressure control.

Sweet Potato / Banana / Almond

~ Sweet Potato - 1.5 cup - boiled - cooled - skin removed - cut into chunks
~ Banana - 2 - peeled - cut in 1 inch pieces - frozen
~ Almonds - 2 tablespoons - sliced
~ Ginger - 1 tablespoon - fresh peeled - slices
~ Turmeric - 1/4 (+-) teaspoon
~ Cinnamon - 1/4 (+-) teaspoon
~ Milk - 1 cup - almond or 2%
~ Water - 1/2 (+-) cup

Sweet Potato / Grapes / Orange / Apple

~ Sweet Potato - 3/4 cup - boiled - cooled - skin removed - cut into chunks
~ Grapes - 1 1/2 cups - red - frozen
~ Orange - 1 medium - peeled - segmented - seeds removed
~ Apple - 1/2 cup - sweet red - cored - peeled - chopped
~ Ginger - 1 tablespoon - fresh peeled - slices
~ Water - 1/4 (+-) cup
~ Ice - 1/4 (+-) cup

Sweet Potato / Romaine Lettuce / Banana / Cashews

~ Sweet Potato - 3/4 cup - boiled - cooled - skin removed - cut into chunks
~ Spinach - 1 1/2 cups - baby - chopped
~ Banana - 1 - peeled - cut in 1 inch pieces - frozen
~ Cashews - 1/4 cup - chopped
~ Cinnamon - 1/4 (+-) teaspoon
~ Vanilla Extract - 1/4 (+-) teaspoon
~ Milk - 1 (+-) cup - 2% or Almond

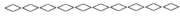

Pumpkin

The pumpkin is a member of the winter squash family. It is high in healthy antioxidants, vitamins, and minerals but low in calories. Although you can cook and prepare fresh pumpkin for your smoothies, all of these recipes call for pre-prepared canned pumpkin. A word of caution, if you buy canned pumpkin make sure it 100% pure pumpkin and not pumpkin pie filling. Also make sure the canned pumpkin does not have added sugars, salt, and/or other preservatives.

Pumpkin / Yogurt / Banana / Orange Juice
~ Pumpkin - 1 cup - canned - chilled
~ Yogurt - 1 cup - unsweetened
~ Banana - 1 - peeled - cut in 1 inch pieces - frozen
~ Orange Juice - 1/2 cup - fresh squeezed
~ Honey - 1 (+-) tablespoon
~ Cinnamon - 1/2 (+-) teaspoon
~ Nutmeg - 1/8 (+-) teaspoon
~ Vanilla Extract - 1/8 (+-) teaspoon
~ Cloves - Dash - to taste
~ Water - 1/4 (+-) cup
~ Ice - 1/2 (+-) cup

Pumpkin / Carrot / Cashew / Grapes
~ Pumpkin - 1 cup - canned - chilled
~ Carrots - 1 cup - chopped
~ Cashews - 1/2 cup - chopped
~ Grapes - 1/2 cup - chopped -frozen
~ Cinnamon - 1 (+-) teaspoon
~ Nutmeg - 1/2 (+-) teaspoon
~ Ginger - 1/4 (+-) teaspoon - ground
~ Cloves - 1/4 (+-) teaspoon - ground
~ Honey - 1 (+-) tablespoon
~ Vanilla Extract - 1/8 (+-) teaspoon
~ Water - 1/2 (+-) cup
~ Ice - 1/2 (+-) cup

(Pumpkin – continued next page)

(Pumpkin – continued)

Pumpkin / Mango / Spinach / Almonds
~ Pumpkin - 1/2 cup - canned - chilled
~ Mango - 1 cup - chunks - frozen
~ Spinach - 1 1/2 cups - baby - chopped
~ Almonds - 3 tablespoons - chopped
~ Vanilla Extract - 1/8 (+-) teaspoon
~ Cinnamon - 1 (+-) teaspoon
~ Milk - 1/2 cup - almond or 2%
~ Water - 1/2 (+-) cup
~ Ice - 4 (+-) cubes
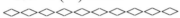

Squash

Squash have been divided into two types, summer squash and winter squash. They were given these designations in a time when what was available at the market was dictated by when it was available from the farms. Now both are usually available in markets year round. Yellow squash and zucchini are the most common summer squash and butternut squash is usually the most common winter squash available year round.

Squash / Blueberry / Orange / Walnut
~ Squash - 1 1/2 cups - yellow - chopped
~ Blueberry - 3/4 cup - frozen
~ Orange - 1 large - peeled - segmented - seeds removed
~ Walnut - 1/4 cup - chopped
~ Water - 1/2 (+-) cup
~ Ice - 1/2 (+-) cup

Squash / Strawberry / Banana / Spinach
~ Squash - 1/2 cup - zucchini - chopped
~ Strawberry - 1 cup - fresh or frozen
~ Banana - 1 - peeled - cut in 1 inch pieces - frozen
~ Spinach - 1 cup - baby - chopped
~ Honey - 1 (+-) tablespoon
~ Water - 1/2 (+-) cup
~ Ice - 1/2 (+-) cup

Squash / Cashew / Orange
~ Squash - 1 cup - butternut - baked - seeds&peel removed - mashed - cooled
~ Cashew - 1/4 cup - chopped
~ Orange - 2 medium - peeled - segmented - seeds removed
~ Milk - 3/4 cup - almond
~ Cinnamon - 1/2 (+-) teaspoon
~ Ginger - 1/4 (+-) teaspoon ground
~ Vanilla Extract - 1/4 (+-) teaspoon
~ Honey - 1 (+-) tablespoon
~ Water - 1/2 (+-) cup
~ Ice - 1/2 (+-) cup

◇◇◇◇◇◇◇◇◇◇

Tomato

Tomatoes come in a variety of sizes, shapes, colors and flavors. Some are tart and others are sweet. Some are very juicy and others have less juice and thicker flesh. Regardless of the variety, the fruit of the tomato plant is one of the world's healthiest foods and filled with vitamins, minerals, and antioxidants.

Tomato / Carrot / Celery
~ Tomato - 2 1/2 cups - chopped
~ Carrot - 1/4 cup - peeled - chopped
~ Celery - 1/4 cup - chopped
~ Lemon - 1/2 medium - peeled - seeds removed
~ Black Pepper - 1/4 (+-) teaspoon
~ Onion Powder - 1/8 (+-) teaspoon - optional to taste
~ Garlic Powder - 1/8 (+-) teaspoon - optional to taste
~ Water - 1/4 (+-) cup
~ Ice - 3/4 (+-) cup

Tomato / Spinach / Mango
~ Tomato - 1 1/2 cups - chopped
~ Spinach - 1 cup - baby - chopped
~ Mango - 3/4 cup - chunks - frozen
~ Basil - 2 (+-) tablespoons - fresh - chopped
~ Water - 1/4 (+-) cup
~ Ice - 3/4 (+-) cup

Tomato / Cantaloupe / Apple / Carrot / Banana
~ Tomato - 1 cup - chopped
~ Cantaloupe - 1 1/2 cups - diced - frozen
~ Apple - 1/4 cup - red - cored - peeled - chopped
~ Carrot - 1/4 cup - peeled - chopped
~ Banana - 1 - peeled - chopped
~ Water - 3/4 (+-) cup
~ Ice - 1/4 (+-) cup
◇◇◇◇◇◇◇◇◇◇

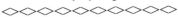

Chapter 6
Smoothie Recipes - Fruits

Many plants commonly considered as vegetables are technically fruits. Cucumber, eggplant, pumpkin, squash, and tomato are examples of fruits commonly referred to as vegetables. All of these are included in the above vegetable section. Colorful and full of flavor, fruits contain many minerals, vitamins, and anti-oxidants that are needed for natural maintenance and control of blood pressure. Most fruits are edible in their raw form and eating them that way usually gives you their maximum nutrition. Many fruits are available in canned form, just make sure that if you use canned fruits that they do not contain added sugars or artificial preservatives. Most fruits can also be dried and in many cases, dried fruit provides a higher concentration per ounce of those nutrients most needed to maintain health blood pressure. If you do use dried fruits just be sure they are prepared without added sweeteners or sulphites. You may also want to re-hydrate dried fruits before using them in your smoothie

Be sure to wash all fresh fruits thoroughly before blending.

Apple

There is a good reason behind the saying "An apple a day keeps the doctor away". Apples are filled with with the flavonoid quercetin which is a powerful antioxidant that helps protect blood vessels from damage and is effective in reducing blood pressure. Apples are also a good source of Vitamin C and Potassium.

Apple / Carrot / Cucumber
~ Apple - 1 cup - sweet variety - cored - with peel - chopped
~ Carrot - 1/2 cup - chopped
~ Cucumber - 1/2 cup - peeled - sliced
~ Apple Juice - 1 cup - organic - no sugar added
~ Water - 1/2 (+-) cup
~ Ice - 1 1/2 (+-) cups
~ Spice - Dash - cinnamon or nutmeg - optional

Apple / Strawberry/ Blueberry / Kiwifruit
~ Apple - 2 - any variety - cored - peeled - chopped
~ Strawberry - 1/2 cup - frozen
~ Blueberry - 1/2 cup - frozen
~ Kiwifruit - 1/2 cup - peel removed
~ Apple Juice - 3/4 (+-) cup - organic - no sugar added
~ Orange Juice - 3/4 (+-) cup - fresh squeezed or organic

Apple / Grape / Spinach
~ Apple - 1 - tart variety - cored - peeled - chopped
~ Grapes - 2 cups - green seedless - frozen
~ Spinach - 1/2 cup - baby - chopped
~ Apple Juice - 1 (+-) cup - organic - no sugar added
~ Water - 1/2 (+-) cup

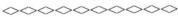

Apricot

Apricots are closely related to peaches and plums, and apricots. They have as much potassium as bananas, and they are a good source of heart healthy antioxidants such as beta-carotene (Vitamin A) and Vitamin C.

Apricot / Mango / Kale / Cashew
~ Apricot - 1 cup - halved - pitted
~ Mango - 1 cup - chunks - frozen
~ Kale - 1/2 cup - chopped
~ Cashew - 1/8 cup - finely chopped
~ Milk - 1 1/2 (+-) cups - almond or 2%

Apricot / Apple/ Strawberry / Spinach / Carrot
~ Apricot - 3/4 cup - halved - pitted
~ Apple - 1/2 cup - sweet variety - cored - with peel - chopped
~ Strawberry - 1/2 cup - frozen
~ Spinach - 1 cup - baby - chopped
~ Carrot - 1/4 cup - peeled - chopped
~ Water - 1/4 (+-) cup
~ Ice - 3/4 (+-) cup

Apricot / Banana / Blueberry
~ Apricot - 1 cup - halved - pitted
~ Banana - 1 large - peeled - cut in 1 inch pieces
~ Blueberry - 1 cup - frozen
~ Milk - 1 (+-) cup - 2% or almond
~ Honey - 2 (+-) teaspoons
~ Water - 1/4 (+-) cup
◇◇◇◇◇◇◇◇◇◇◇

Avocado

The avocado has a high fat content but it is a monounsaturated fat not the unhealthy types (trans fat and refined polyunsaturated fat) that are found in most processed foods. Some studies show when eaten with other foods, the type of fat found in the avocado increases vitamin and antioxidant absorption from those other foods. Avocados are a great source for potassium since they contain a lot more of it than bananas. Be sure to always remove and discard the large pit from the avocado before using.

Avocado / Watermelon / Banana / Orange Juice

~ Avocado - 1 cup - pitted - peeled - chopped
~ Watermelon - 1 cup - chunks - frozen
~ Banana - 1 medium - peeled - cut in 1 inch pieces
~ Orange Juice - 1 (+-) cup - fresh squeezed
~ Water - 1/4 (+-) cup

Avocado / Cucumber / Grapes

~ Avocado - 2 cups - pitted - peeled - chopped
~ Cucumber - 1/2 cup - peeled - chopped
~ Grapes - 1/2 cup - green - seedless - frozen
~ Yogurt - 1/2 cup - plain - low-fat
~ Milk - 1/4 (+-) cup - 2% or low-fat
~ Honey - 1 (+-) teaspoons
~ Ice - 1/4 (+-) cup

Avocado / Strawberry / Lemon

~ Avocado - 2 cups - pitted - peeled - chopped
~ Strawberry - 1 cup - frozen
~ Lemon - 1/2 medium - juiced - use juice only
~ Milk - 1 (+-) cup
~ Honey - 1 (+-) teaspoons
~ Water - 1/4 (+-) cup

◇◇◇ ◇◇◇◇◇◇

Banana

Because of its high potassium content, the first fruit that comes to mind when thinking about blood pressure control is the banana. Bananas are consumed in almost all countries in the world. Once a banana is ripe, it can peeled then sliced, chopped, pureed, or placed whole in a freezer bag and frozen. They can be stored this way in a freezer for about 2 months. If you add lemon juice to the bananas before freezing, it will help prevent discoloration. Many of the smoothie recipes in this book that call for bananas specify that they be sliced and frozen. This gives a chill to the smoothie without having to add more ice. Use very ripe bananas in smoothies to get the best taste.

Banana / Vanilla Yogurt
~ Banana - 2 medium - peeled - cut in 1 inch pieces
~ Yogurt - 1 cup - vanilla - non-fat
~ Milk - 1/2 (+-) cup - 2% or low fat
~ Ice - 1 (+-) cup

Banana / Apple
~ Banana - 2 medium - peeled - cut in 1 inch pieces - frozen
~ Apple - 1 medium - sweet red - peeled - cored - chopped
~ Milk - 1 (+-) cup - almond, 2%, or low-fat
~ Nutmeg - 1 pinch to taste (optional)

Banana / Spinach / Mango / Pomegranate
~ Banana - 1 medium - peeled - cut in 1 inch pieces
~ Spinach - 1 cup - chopped - frozen
~ Mango - 1/2 cup - chunks - frozen
~ Pomegranate - 1/2 cup - arils or juice
~ Milk - 1 (+-) cup - almond, 2%, or low-fat
~ Honey - 1 (+-) teaspoon
◇◇◇◇◇◇◇◇◇◇◇

Berries

Since prehistoric times, wild berries have been a food source for humans. Domesticated varieties of berries are filled with varying amounts of anti-oxidants, vitamins and/or minerals. The three listed here (blackberry, blueberry, and strawberry) are filled with those nutrients needed for healthy blood pressure control. Berries come in many colors and the high anti-oxidant content of berries come from the chemicals that give berries their colors.

Blackberry / Apple / Kale
~ Blackberry - 1 cups - unsweetened - frozen
~ Apple - 1 medium - unpeeled - cored - chopped
~ Kale - 2 cups - fresh baby
~ Water - 1/2 (+-) cup

Blueberry / Yogurt
~ Blueberry - 2 cups - unsweetened - frozen
~ Yogurt - 1 cup - plain - unsweetened
~ Milk - 1 (+-) cup - 2%, low-fat, or almond
~ Honey - 1 (+-) teaspoon

Strawberry / Cantaloupe
~ Strawberry - 1 1/2 cups - unsweetened - frozen
~ Cantaloupe - 1 cup - peeled - chunks
~ Milk - 1 1/2 (+-) cup - 2%, or low-fat
~ Vanilla Extract - 1/2 (+-) teaspoon
~ Ice - 3 (+-) cubes

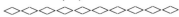

Fig

Fresh figs have a shelf live of only a few days. Dried figs have a much longer shelf life and drying figs greatly increases the mineral concentration per cup of figs. If kept in a cool, dark place, or in the refrigerator, dried figs have a shelf life of up to several months. You can re-hydrate dried figs to make them juicer and easier to use in making a smoothie. It is best to soak dried figs for 8 to 12 hours in water or milk before using them in a smoothie.

Fig / Cucumber / Orange
~ Figs - 3/4 cup - fresh or re-hydrated dried - chopped
~ Cucumber - 1 cup - peeled - chopped - frozen
~ Orange - 1 large - peeled - segmented - seeds removed
~ Milk - 1 (+-) cup - 2% or Almond

Fig / Mango / Kale / Lemon
~ Figs - 1 cup - fresh or re-hydrated dried - chopped
~ Mango - 3/4 cup - chunks - frozen
~ Kale - 1 cup - baby - chopped
~ Lemon - 1/2 medium - peeled - seeds removed
~ Milk - 1 (+-) cup - 2% or Almond
~ Honey - 1 (+-) tablespoon
~ Ice - 1/4 (+-) cup

Fig / Yogurt / walnut
~ Figs - 1 3/4 cup - fresh or re-hydrated dried - chopped
~ Yogurt - 1 1/2 cup - vanilla - low-fat
~ Walnut - 1/4 cup - finely chopped
~ Milk - 1/2 (+-) cup - 2% or Almond
~ Cinnamon - 1/4 (+-) teaspoon
~ Vanilla extract - 1/4 (+-) teaspoon

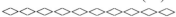

Kiwifruit

The kiwifruit has a peel that is a fuzzy brownish/green, a shape and size that resembles a chicken egg, and an inside flesh that is bright green with tiny black seed around the core. The kiwifruit is a great source of heart healthy minerals, antioxidants, and omega-3 fatty acids. A cup of sliced kiwifruit has a lot more Vitamin C, potassium, and magnesium than a cup of orange sections.

Kiwi / Banana / Blueberry
~ Kiwi - 1 cup - peeled - sliced
~ Banana - 1 medium - peeled - cut in 1 inch pieces - frozen
~ Blueberry - 3/4 cup - frozen
~ Yogurt - 1 cup - vanilla - non-fat
~ Water - 1/4 (+-) cup
~ Vanilla Extract - 1/8 (+-) teaspoon (optional)

Kiwi / Cucumber / Apple
~ Kiwi - 1 cup - peeled - sliced
~ Cucumber - 3/4 cup - peeled - chopped - frozen
~ Apple - 3/4 cup - any variety - cored - peeled
~ Milk - 1 (+-) cup - almond, 2% , or low-fat
~ Ice - 1/2 (+-) cup

Kiwi / Mango / Broccoli / Cauliflower
~ Kiwi - 3/4 cup - peeled - sliced
~ Mango - 3/4 cup - chunks - frozen
~ Broccoli - 1 cup - chopped - frozen
~ Cauliflower - 1/2 cup - chopped
~ Water - 1 (+-) cup
◇◇◇◇◇◇◇◇◇◇◇

Mango

Mango is known as the "king of fruits" and is one of the most commonly eaten fruit in the tropical countries of the world. Its sweet, juicy, orange-yellow flesh is rich in vitamins, minerals, and antioxidants. Fully ripened mangoes in sliced, cubed, or chunk form can be stored in airtight containers in a freezer for 6 to 10 months.

Mango / Orange
~ Mango - 2 cups - chunks - frozen
~ Orange - 1 cup - peeled - segmented - seeds removed
~ Orange Juice - 1 cup - fresh squeezed

Mango / Carrot / Apple
~ Mango - 1 1/2 cups - chunks - frozen
~ Carrot - 1 cup - peeled - chopped
~ Apple - 1/2 cup - any variety - cored - peeled
~ Honey - 1 (+-) tablespoon
~ Apple Juice - 1/2 (+-) cup - unsweetened
~ Water - 1/2 (+-) cup - unsweetened

Mango / Banana / Kale
~ Mango - 1 1/2 cups - chunks - fresh or frozen
~ Banana - 1 medium - peeled - cut in 1 inch pieces - frozen
~ Kale - 1/2 cup - fresh baby - chopped
~ Vanilla Extract - 1 (+-) teaspoon
~ Milk - 3/4 cup - 2%, low-fat, or almond
~ Ice - 1/4 (+-) cup

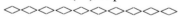

Melon - Cantaloupe

Aside from the watermelon, the cantaloupe is one of the two most readily available melons in US markets. The cantaloupe has an edible sweet orangish flesh inside its rind. The cantaloupe is mostly water but it is nutrient filled with heart healthy minerals and vitamins.

Cantaloupe / Cucumber / Orange

~ Cantaloupe - 2 cups - rind and seeds removed - chunks - frozen
~ Cucumber - 1/2 cup - peeled - chopped
~ Orange - 1/2 cup - peeled - segmented - seeds removed
~ Yogurt - 1/2 cup - unsweetened - nonfat or low-fat
~ Orange Juice - 1/2 cup - fresh squeezed
~ Honey - 1 (+-) teaspoon
~ Vanilla Extract - 1/2 (+-) teaspoon

Cantaloupe / Grape / Tomato / Carrot

~ Cantaloupe - 1 cup - rind and seeds removed - chunks - frozen
~ Grape - 3/4 cup - red or purple - seedless - frozen
~ Tomato - 1 medium - chopped
~ Carrot - 1/2 cup - baby - chopped
~ Honey - 1 (+-) teaspoon
~ Water - 1 (+-) cup

Cantaloupe / Strawberry / Banana / Almond

~ Cantaloupe - 1 1/2 cup - rind and seeds removed - chunks
~ Strawberry - 1 cup - frozen
~ Banana - 1 medium - peeled - cut in 1 inch pieces
~ Almond - 1/4 cup - chopped
~ Honey - 1 (+-) teaspoon
~ Milk - 1/2 (+-) 2%, low-fat, almond

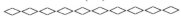

Melon - Honeydew

The honeydew melon is also one of the two most readily available melons (not counting watermelon) in US markets. The honeydew melon has an edible sweet creamy/white flesh inside its rind. Like the cantaloupe, the honeydew is mostly water but it is also nutrient filled with heart healthy minerals and vitamins.

Honeydew / Yogurt / Apple Juice
~ Honeydew - 2 cups - rind and seeds removed - chunks - frozen
~ Yogurt - 1 cup - vanilla - low-fat
~ Apple Juice - 1 (+-) cup - unsweetened

Honeydew / Blueberry / Zucchini / Lemon
~ Honeydew - 1 1/2 cups - rind and seeds removed - chunks
~ Blueberry - 1 cup - frozen
~ Zucchini - 1 cup - frozen
~ Lemon - 1/2 medium - juice only
~ Water - 1/2 (+-) cup

Honeydew / Spinach / Strawberry
~ Honeydew - 1 3/4 cups - rind and seeds removed - chunks
~ Spinach - 1 cup - frozen
~ Strawberry - 1 cup - frozen - no sugar added
~ Water - 1/4 (+-) cup

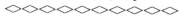

Orange

Today, the orange is probably the world's most popular citrus fruit but that only became possible in America during the 20th century when advances in processing and transportation allowed year round consumption of oranges practical. The World Health Organization recently issued a report that said that because of the citrus fruit's high levels of potassium as well as vitamin C, carotenoids, and flavonoids, a diet that includes citrus fruits offers protection against cardiovascular disease.

Orange / Yogurt
~ Orange - 2 cups - peeled - segmented - seeds removed - frozen
~ Yogurt - 1 cup - vanilla - low-fat
~ Orange Juice - 1/4 (+-) cup - fresh squeezed
~ Honey - 1 (+-) tablespoon
~ Vanilla Extract - 1/2 (+-) teaspoon
~ Ice - 1/2 (+-) cup

Orange / Kale / Banana / Cucumber / Ginger
~ Orange - 1 cups - peeled - segmented - seeds removed
~ Kale - 1/2 cup - fresh baby - chopped
~ Banana - 1 medium - peeled - cut in 1 inch pieces - frozen
~ Cucumber - 1/2 cup - peeled - chopped - frozen
~ Ginger Root - 1/2 (+-) inch piece - finely chopped
~ Water - 1/2 (+-) cup

Orange / Apricot
~ Orange - 1 cups - peeled - segmented - seeds removed
~ Apricot - 1 cups - fresh or re-hydrated dried - chopped
~ Yogurt - 1/2 cup - unsweetened - low-fat
~ Orange Juice - 1/4 (+-) cup - fresh squeezed
~ Honey - 1 (+-) tablespoon
~ Ice - 1 1/2 (+-) cup

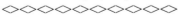

Pomegranate

The sweet-tart flavor of pomegranates makes them a favorite ingredient in many recipes. Pomegranates have high levels of antioxidants along with high amounts of potassium and magnesium. This is what gives pomegranates their blood pressure reducing properties. The outer skin of the pomegranate is tough and not eaten. The edible parts of the pomegranate are the seed (called arils) and the white pithy part surrounding the seeds. Note: take care when cutting and removing seeds from a pomegranate. Pomegranate juice can stain clothes, wood cutting boards, porous counter-tops, wood cooking utensils, etc...

Pomegranate / Strawberry / Cucumber
~ Pomegranate - 1 ripe - cut - arils only
~ Strawberry - 1 cup - unsweetened - frozen
~ Cucumber - 1/2 cup - peeled - chopped - frozen
~ Yogurt - 1 cup - vanilla - low-fat
~ Milk - 1/4 (+-) cup - 2%, low-fat, or almond
~ Water - 1/4 (+-) cup

Pomegranate / Mango / Kale
~ Pomegranate - 1 ripe - cut - arils only
~ Mango - 1 1/2 cups - chunks - frozen
~ Kale - 1 cup - fresh baby
~ Milk - 1/2 (+-) cup - 2%, low-fat, or almond

Pomegranate / Banana / Cashew
~ Pomegranate Juice - 1 cup - unsweetened
~ Banana - 2 large - peeled - sliced - frozen
~ Cashew - 1/4 cup - unsalted - chopped
~ Milk - 3/4 (+-) cup - 2%, low-fat, or almond
~ Honey - 2 (+-) tablespoons
◇◇◇◇◇◇◇◇◇◇◇

Prune

When you say prunes, almost everyone knows what they are, but many don't realize that prunes are just dried plums. To get a wider market for their product, many suppliers are changing the name of their product from prunes to dried plums. By either name, the end product is still the same. Like most other fruits, dried plums contain a higher concentration of the vitamins and minerals needed for healthy blood pressure than the fresh plum. The main exception to this is that vitamin the C content is higher in a fresh fruit than in the dried version. Prunes are usually made from the large bluish purple plum. If you buy prepackaged prunes (dried plums), make sure that the pits have been removed and that no sugars, preservatives, and/or other additives have been used.

For the recipes that call for re-hydrated prunes, put the prunes in hot water for about 15 minutes. Once plump, drain, and let the plums cool before using in a smoothie.

Prunes / Banana / Spinach
~ Prunes - 6 re-hydrated - pits removed - chopped
~ Banana - 1 medium - peeled - cut in 1 inch pieces - frozen
~ Spinach - 1 1/2 cup - fresh baby - chopped
~ Milk - 1 (+-) cup - 2%, low-fat - almond
~ Ice - 1/2 (+-) cup
~ Honey - 2 (+-) tablespoons

Prune Juice / Carrot / Celery / Apple
~ Prune Juice - 1 cup - unsweetened
~ Carrot - 1/2 cup - baby - chopped - frozen
~ Celery - 1/2 cup - chopped - frozen
~ Apple - 1 medium - sweet red - cored - peeled - seeds removed
~ Orange Juice - 1/2 cup - fresh squeezed
~ Ice - 1/2 (+-) cup

(Prunes – continued next page)

(Prunes – continued)

Prunes / Apple Juice / Yogurt
~ Prunes - 6 re-hydrated - pits removed - chopped
~ Apple Juice - 1 1/2 cups - unsweetened
~ Yogurt - 1 cup - vanilla - low-fat
~ Cinnamon - 1/8 (+-)
~ Vanilla Extract - 3/4 (+-)
~ Nutmeg - 1 (+-) pinch (optional to taste)
~ Ice - 1/2 (+-) cup
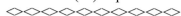

Raisins

Raisins are dried grapes. Raisins are like prunes (dried plums) in that, except for vitamin C, dried raisins have a higher concentration of the vitamins and minerals needed for healthy blood pressure than the same volume of fresh grapes. Although consumed around the world, about half of the world's supply of raisins are grown in California.

Like with prunes, for the recipes that call for re-hydrated raisins, put the raisins in hot water for about 15 minutes. Once plump, drain, and let them cool before using in a smoothie.

Raisin / Apple
~ Raisin - 1/2 cup - re-hydrated
~ Apple - 1 medium - any variety - cored - seeds removed - chopped
~ Milk - 1 1/2 cups - 2%, low-fat, almond
~ Cinnamon - 1/4 (+-) teaspoon
~ Vanilla Extract - 1/2 (+-) tablespoon
~ Ice - 1 (+-) cup

Raisin / Banana / Strawberry
~ Raisin - 1/4 cup - re-hydrated
~ Banana - 1 medium - peeled - cut in 1 inch pieces - frozen
~ Strawberry - 1 cup - unsweetened - frozen
~ Yogurt - 1 1/2 cup - vanilla - low-fat
~ Oats - 4 tablespoons - uncooked quick oats
~ Milk - 1/2 (+-) cups - 2%, low-fat, or almond
~ Honey - 1 (+-) tablespoon
~ Cinnamon - 1/4 (+-) teaspoon

Raisin - Kale - Cucumber
~ Raisin - 1/4 cup - re-hydrated
~ Kale - 1 cup - fresh baby - chopped
~ Cucumber - 1 cup - peeled - chopped - frozen
~ Yogurt - 1 cup - plain - low-fat
~ Grape Juice - 3/4 (+-) cups - white - unsweetened
~ Ice - 1/4 (+-) cup

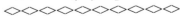

Watermelon

Watermelons come in many colors both inside (inner flesh) and out (rind). They can have seeds or be seedless, and come in sizes from very small to very large. All parts of a watermelon are edible, including the seeds and the rind. There are nutrients that help with blood pressure control in the watermelon flesh, the seeds, and the rind. Just be sure to wash the rind thoroughly before consuming.

Watermelon / Honey
~ Watermelon - 3 cups - rind and seeds removed - cubed - frozen
~ Honey - 2 (+-) teaspoons
~ Basil - 1 (+-) teaspoon (optional to taste) - fresh sweet - chopped
~ Water - 1 (+-) cup

Watermelon / Blueberry
~ Watermelon - 1 1/2 cups - rind and seeds removed - cubed
~ Blueberry - 1 cup - unsweetened - frozen
~ Yogurt - 1 cup - plain - low-fat
~ Honey - 2 (+-) teaspoons (optional)
~ Milk - 1/4 (+-) cup - 2%, low-fat, or almond
~ Ice - 1/4 (+-) cup

Watermelon / Mango

~ Watermelon - 2 cups - rind and seeds removed - cubed
~ Mango - 1 cup - chunks - frozen
~ Water - 1/2 (+-) cup
~ Ice - 1/2 (+-) cup
◇◇◇◇◇◇◇◇◇◇

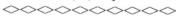

Chapter 7
Smoothie Recipes - Beans

Beans are high in protein and are another rich source of needed vitamins and minerals. Beans have been used as meat substitutes in many diets and recipes for thousands of years. The many varieties of beans are great additions to an economical and nutritious diet. For recipes to include in this book, I used the most common types of beans consumed in America. The ones selected are highest in the three important minerals needed for effective blood pressure control (potassium, magnesium, and calcium). The recipes I included are for black beans, kidney beans, pinto beans, and soybeans.

Beans can be purchased fresh, frozen, canned, or dried. If you use canned beans be sure to get low or no sodium added brands. Also be sure they have no added sugars or artificial preservatives. For canned beans that do contain sodium, rinse them before using to remove as much of the added sodium as possible.

Black Bean / Cucumber / Blueberry / Spinach
~ Black Bean - 1/2 cup - cooked - cooled
~ Cucumber - 1 cup - peeled - chopped
~ Blueberry - 1 cup - unsweetened - frozen
~ Spinach - 1 cup - frozen
~ Honey - 1 (+-) tablespoon
~ Water - 1/2 (+-) cup

Kidney Bean / Mango / Strawberry / Walnut
~ Kidney Bean - 1/2 cup - cooked - cooled
~ Mango - 1 cup - unsweetened - frozen
~ Strawberry - 1 cup - unsweetened - frozen
~ Walnut - 1/4 (+-) cup - chopped
~ Sweet Basil - 1 (+-) tablespoon - fresh chopped
~ Milk - 1 (+-) cup - 2%, low-fat, almond

Pinto Bean / Blackberry / Pumpkin

~ Pinto Bean - 1 1/2 cups - canned - drained - rinsed
~ Blackberry - 1 cup - unsweetened - frozen
~ Pumpkin - 1/2 cup - canned
~ Yogurt - 1 cup - plain - low-fat
~ Milk - 1/4 (+-) cup - 2%, low-fat, almond

Soybean / Carrot / Strawberry / Apple

~ Soybean - 1 cup - Edamame - frozen
~ Carrot - 1/2 cup - baby - chopped
~ Strawberry - 1 cup - unsweetened - frozen
~ Apple - 1 medium - sweet - cored - seeds removed - chopped
~ Milk - 1/2 (+-) cup - 2%, low-fat, almond

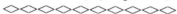

Chapter 8
Smoothie Recipes - Nuts

The American Heart Association recommends four to five servings of nuts a week. Many types of nuts are good sources of potassium and magnesium and some are also good sources of healthy Omega-3 fat. For high blood pressure control, you should only eat nuts either raw or dry roasted. Nuts roasted in hydrogenated oils usually have added salt and both of these cause increases in blood pressure. It is important that you don't go overboard in your daily consumption of nuts since they are usually high in calories and some contain unhealthy Omega-6 fats. As I did with beans, I have included recipes for the most common types of nuts consumed in America and that are highest in the three important minerals needed for effective blood pressure control (potassium, magnesium, and calcium). I have included the top five: almonds, Brazil nut, cashews, pistachio, and walnuts. All of these are tree nuts. Even though they have beneficial nutrients, I did not include peanuts (a legume not a tree nut) because peanuts have a high level of omega-6 fatty acids and because the high prevalence of peanut allergies in today's population.

Note: For softer nuts to use in smoothies, put the nuts in a container, fill the container with cold water and soak at least 1 hour. If you soak them longer keep the container with nuts and water in the refrigerator until ready to use. Drain after soaking and before using in smoothie.

Almond / Blueberry
~ Almonds - 1/4 cup - raw or dry roasted - unsalted -chopped
~ Blueberry - 1 1/2 cups - unsweetened - fresh or frozen
~ Honey - 2 (+-) tablespoons
~ Milk - 1 1/4 cup - 2%, low-fat, or almond
~ Ice - 1 (+-) cup

Brazil Nut / Banana / Yogurt
~ Brazil Nut - 1/4 cup - raw - soaked overnight - unsalted -chopped
~ Banana - 2 medium - peeled - cut in 1 inch pieces - frozen
~ Yogurt - 1 cup - unsweetened - low-fat
~ Vanilla Extract - 1 (+-) teaspoon
~ Honey - 1 (+-) teaspoon
~ Milk - 3/4 (+-) cup - 2%, low-fat, or almond
~ Ice - 1/2 (+-) cup

Cashew / Apple / Mango / Spinach
~ Cashew - 1/4 cup - raw - soaked overnight - unsalted -chopped
~ Apple - 1 small - sweet red - cored - peeled - seeds removed - chopped
~ Mango - 1 cup - unsweetened - frozen
~ Spinach - 1 1/2 cup - frozen
~ Honey - 1 (+-) teaspoon
~ Cinnamon - 1 (+-) teaspoon
~ Nutmeg - 1/4 (+-) teaspoon
~ Water - 1/4 (+-) cup

Pistachio / Cantaloupe / Celery
~ Pistachio - 1/4 cup - raw or dry roasted - unsalted -chopped
~ Cantaloupe - 1 cup - peeled - chunks - frozen
~ Celery - 1/2 cup - finely chopped - frozen
~ Yogurt - 1 cup - unsweetened - low-fat
~ Milk - 3/4 (+-) cup - 2%, low-fat, or almond
~ Honey - 2 (+-) tablespoons

Walnut / Avocado / Strawberry / Apple
~ Walnut - 1/4 cup - raw - unsalted -chopped
~ Avocado - 1 cup - pitted - peeled - chopped
~ Strawberry - 1 cup - unsweetened - frozen
~ Apple - 1 medium - sweet - cored - seeds removed - chopped
~ Milk - 1 (+-) cup - 2%, low-fat, or almond
~ Vanilla Extract - 1/2 (+-) teaspoon
~ Honey - 1 (+-) teaspoon

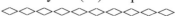

Chapter 9
Smoothie Recipes - Herbs and Spice

Used to enhance the flavor of foods and to make eating more pleasurable, herbs and spices are added to all sorts of recipes. Herbs and spices have also been used since prehistoric times for their medicinal properties. In this chapter I have listed the familiar herbs and spices that can have beneficial effects in maintaining a healthy blood pressure level. These are basil, black pepper, ginger, oregano, and turmeric.

Basil / Zucchini / Strawberry
~ Basil - 2 teaspoons - fresh - finely chopped
~ Zucchini - 1 cup - chopped - frozen
~ Strawberry - 2 cups - unsweetened - frozen
~ Honey - 1 (+-) tablespoon
~ Water - 1 (+-) cup

Black Pepper / Watermelon / Orange
~ Black Pepper - 1 tablespoon / course ground -
~ Watermelon - 2 cups - rind and seeds removed - chopped - frozen
~Orange - 1 medium - peeled - segmented - seeds removed
~ Yogurt - 1 cup - vanilla - low-fat
~ Orange Juice - 1/2 (+-) cup - fresh squeezed

Ginger / Mango / Apricot / Bok Choy
~ Ginger - 1 inch piece -fresh root- finely minced
~ Mango - 1 1/2 cup - unsweetened - frozen
~ Apricot - 1 cup - halved - pitted - unsweetened - frozen
~ Bok Choy - 1 cup - leaves and stalks - chopped
~ Lemon Juice - 1/4 cup - fresh squeezed
~ Water - 3/4 (+-) cup

Oregano / Tomato / Carrot / Cucumber / Garlic
~ Oregano - 1 tablespoon - ground
~ Tomato - 1 cup - chopped
~ Carrot - 1 cup - baby - chopped - frozen
~ Cucumber - 1/2 cup - peeled - chopped - frozen
~ Garlic - 1 clove - minced
~ Water - 1/2 (+-) cup
~ Ice - 1/2 (+-) cup

Turmeric / Banana / Blueberry
~ Turmeric - 1/4 teaspoon - ground
~ Banana - 2 large - peeled - cut in 1 inch pieces - frozen
~ Blueberry - 1 cup - unsweetened - frozen
~ Milk - 1 1/4 cup - 2%, low-fat, or almond
~ Lemon Juice - 1/4 (+-) cup - fresh squeezed

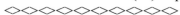

Chapter 10
Smoothie Recipes - Other

I am listing items in this section that did not exactly fit in any of the above categories but are items that I personally am using in my effort to reduce and maintain a healthy blood pressure level. The three items in this chapter are hibiscus tea, lemons, and olive oil.

Hibiscus Tea

In clinical human studies, hibiscus tea was shown to lower blood pressure and speed up metabolism. Hibiscus tea has a much higher antioxidant content than green tea and it also has anti-inflammatory effects.

Hibiscus / Strawberry / Blackberry / Orange
~ Hibiscus Tea - 1 cup - strong brewed - cooled
~ Strawberry - 1 cup - unsweetened - frozen
~ Blackberry - 1 cup - unsweetened - frozen
~ Orange - 1 large - peeled - segmented - seeds removed
~ Honey - 1 (+-) tablespoon

Hibiscus / Blueberry / Cucumber
~ Hibiscus Tea - 2 cups - strong brewed - cooled
~ Blueberry - 1 cup - unsweetened - frozen
~ Cucumber - 1 cup - peeled - chopped - frozen
~ Honey - 1 (+-) tablespoon

Hibiscus / Banana
~ Hibiscus Tea - 1 3/4 cups - strong brewed - cooled
~ Banana - 2 cups - peeled - cut in 1 inch pieces - frozen
~ Water - 1/4 (+-) cup
~ Honey - 1 (+-) tablespoon
◇◇◇◇◇◇◇◇◇◇◇

Lemon

Lemons are a citris fruit high in vitamin C (a powerful anti-oxidant) and help lower blood pressure by helping to keep blood vessels pliable and soft.

Lemon / Blackberry / Yogurt
~ Lemon - 2 medium - washed thoroughly - sliced - seeds removed
~ Blackberry - 1 cup - unsweetened - frozen
~ Yogurt - 1 1/2 cups - vanilla - low-fat
~ Honey - 3 (+-) tablespoons
~ Ice - 1/2 (+-) cup

Lemon / Strawberry / Orange / Banana
~ Lemon - 1 medium - peeled - sliced - seeds removed
~ Strawberry - 1 cup - unsweetened - frozen
~ Orange - 1 cup - peeled - segmented
~ Banana - 1 medium - peeled - cut in 1 inch pieces - frozen
~ Milk - 1 (+-) cup - 2%, low-fat, or almond
~ Honey - 1 (+-) tablespoon

Lemon / Mango / Yogurt
~ Lemon Juice - 1/4 cup - fresh squeezed
~ Mango - 2 cups - chunks - frozen
~ Yogurt - 1 cup - vanilla - low-fat
~ Milk - 3/4 (+-) cup - 2%, low-fat, or almond
~ Vanilla Extract - 1 (+-) teaspoon

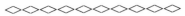

Olive Oil

Like the fatty acids in fish, olive oil contains omega-3 fatty acids. These acids are not produced in the body but are considered essential for human health.

Olive Oil - Strawberry / Cucumber / Kiwi
~ Olive Oil - 1 tablespoon
~ Strawberry - 1 cup - unsweetened - frozen
~ Cucumber - 1 cup - peeled - sliced - frozen
~ Kiwi - 3/4 cup - peeled - sliced
~ Vanilla Extract - 1 (+-) teaspoon
~ Honey - 1 (+-) tablespoon

Olive Oil / Mango / Bok Choy / Carrot
~ Olive Oil - 1 tablespoon
~ Mango - 2 cups - chunks - frozen
~ Bok Choy - 1 cup - leaves and stalks - chopped
~ Carrot - 1/2 cup - baby - chopped
~ Orange Juice - 1/2 (+-) cup - fresh squeezed
~ Lemon Juice - 1/4 (+-) cup - fresh squeezed

Olive Oil / Avocado / Spinach / Banana
~ Olive Oil - 2 tablespoons
~ Avocado - 1/2 cup - peeled - pitted - chopped
~ Spinach - 1 cup - frozen

~ Banana - 1 large - peeled - cut in 1 inch pieces - frozen
~ Yogurt - 1 cup - plain - low-fat
~ Honey - 1 (+-) tablespoon
~ Basil - 1 (+-) tablespoon (optional to taste)
~ Water - 1/2 (+-) cup

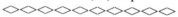

Chapter 11
Last Words

I have listed 125 recipes in this book, but there are thousands of delicious combinations that can be made from using the ingredients included in different recipe categories. I hope you have found several recipes you like in this book but feel free to try your own combinations depending on your individual tastes. The goal is to get the healthy nutrients you need to help reduce and/or control high blood pressure. A good place to start is to pick one item from the Vegetables or Beans category, two items from the Fruits category, and a liquid like water or milk. To make the smoothie sweeter, pick naturally sweet fruits like mango or banana, or add honey. To make it less sweet, add more vegetable items like leafy greens, tomatoes, or beans. For variety try adding unsalted crushed item from the Nuts category and/or some of the items from the Herbs & Spice or Other categories. If you make a bad tasting smoothie, don't let that stop you from trying other combinations. As I said earlier in this book, once you find a combination you like, the more likely you are to make and drink it on a regular basis. Once you make drinking a smoothie every day a habit, the more you will reap the benefits of maintaining a healthy diet.

To help you with creating your own special smoothie combination, I have included on the next page a list of the featured items from all the categories included in this book.

Vegetables & Beans

* Asparagus, * Bok Choy, * Broccoli, * Brussel sprouts, * Cabbage, * Carrots, * Celery, * Cauliflower, * Cucumber, * Eggplant, * Fennel, * Garlic, * Leafy Greens, * Onion, * Potatoes, * Potatoes – Sweet, * Pumpkin, * Squash, * Tomatoes, * Black Bean, * Kidney Bean, * Pinto Bean, * Soybean

Fruits

* Apples, * Apricots, * Avocado, * Banana, * Berries, * Figs, * Kiwifruit, * Mango, * Melon-Cantaloupe, * Melon-Honeydew, * Oranges, * Pomegranate, * Prunes, * Raisins, * Watermelon

Nuts

* Almonds, * Brazil Nut, * Cashews, * Pistachio, * Walnuts

Herbs and Spice

* Basil, * Black Pepper, * Ginger, * Oregano, * Turmeric

Other

* Hibiscus Tea, * Lemons, * Olive Oil

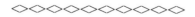

On a personal note, I have been able to achieve a marked blood pressure reduction by following the natural methods of blood pressure control presented in my book High Blood Pressure and You - The Effects of High Blood Pressure, Prescription Drug Side Effects, and Natural Ways To Reduce And Control High Blood Pressure. The results from following these methods were good enough that I was able to stop taking prescription medication for high blood pressure. One of these methods (and one that I really like) is increasing my consumption of healthy nutrients by making and drinking smoothies. I hope you try many of these recipes and find many that you really like. Once you find those combination you like, it will be easier to add drinking smoothies as a healthy habit and you will start feeling the effects of having a healthier lifestyle.

"Knowledge is of no value unless you put it into practice." ~ Anton Chekhov

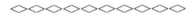

Disclaimer:

END

Notes

Notes

_____

_____

_____

_____

_____

_____

_____

_____

_____

_____

_____

_____

_____

_____

_____

_____

_____

_____

_____